DEDICATION

I dedicate this book to all parents who just want what is best for their kids and their family. May this book be a helpful guide in preparing meals and snacks as part of your daily routine.

Table of Contents

Chapter 1 - Introduction

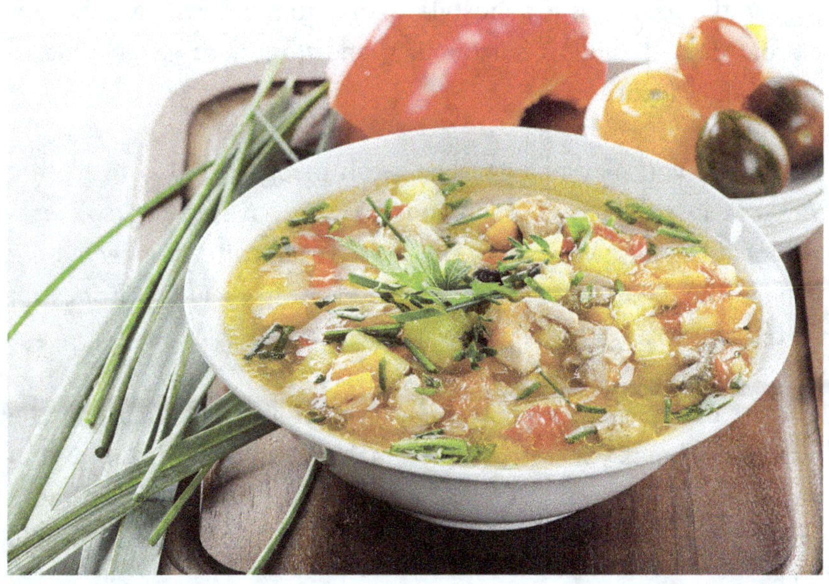

A lifestyle that is healthy and promotes a good quality of life is important. As a parent, it is also one of the best gifts you can give to your children. Food is a necessity for our bodies to thrive but we live in a society were eating habits have moved in the wrong direction.

A lack of time, a lack of information, and the availability of processed foods has resulted in obesity, increased health risks, and reduced lifespan. These negative outcomes can make life difficult due to reduced energy, not being as alert, and an array of potential health problems.

If you are interested in making positive changes for yourself and for your household, consider the gluten free living option. You may be saying you are too busy for gluten free diet programs or that you will be limited in the foods you can buy.

However, this doesn't have to be the case. There are plenty of recipes and variety that are easy to make. There are more restaurants and grocery stores today that offer gluten free options than in the past. This is a lifestyle change that you will find there is a great deal of support surrounding and that makes it possible to successfully incorporate.

Until now, you may not have paid too much attention to gluten. Yet it is in so many of the foods that the average person eats without thinking twice about doing so. It seems to be everywhere you look now that you are making the effort to exclude it from your diet.

Instead of focusing on that negative fact though, focus on the positive changes you are going to make and the opportunity that you have to improve your overall well-being. As you learn more about gluten free products you can make better choices that help you.

Initially, a gluten free lifestyle may seem too hard to implement, but it doesn't have to be. Here, you will get the information you need about why you can live healthier and happier with this type of diet. You will find out methods for shopping and eating out that make it easier.

By eliminating the myths and sticking to the facts you can formulate your plan of action. You will get information about recipes, support, and the health benefits. As you read through the materials, you will be motivated to embrace such changes and you will have the methods to do so!

Not everyone out there is ready to act with a gluten free diet, and that is okay. Freedom of choice is very important. If you feel it is right for you than don't worry about what other people think. If you are friendly as you explain your reasons and while talking to those in a restaurant that are serving you then it isn't out of line at all.

In 2010, various research companies including the National Restaurant Association and American Culinary Federation named gluten free as one of the top food priorities to consider for their establishments. They realized this was more than a passing trend.

For millions of people, it has become a lifestyle choice that they engage in every single day. Are you ready to join them? It seems like all of the doors are wide open at this point when it comes to overall opportunity. The barriers that used to be in place such as limited products that were gluten free and a lack of information have been slowly removed.

Gluten problems can affect people of all ages, including children. There is no indication that any race or gender is more likely to be affected by it than others. The sooner that the problem is identified though the better.

Many adults develop this problem as they get older and there are a multitude of reasons why. There is nothing you can do to prevent it though as it is a genetic factor. You can take action though to live a good quality of life though in spite of the situation.

Chapter 2- What Do You Mean By Gluten Free Diet?

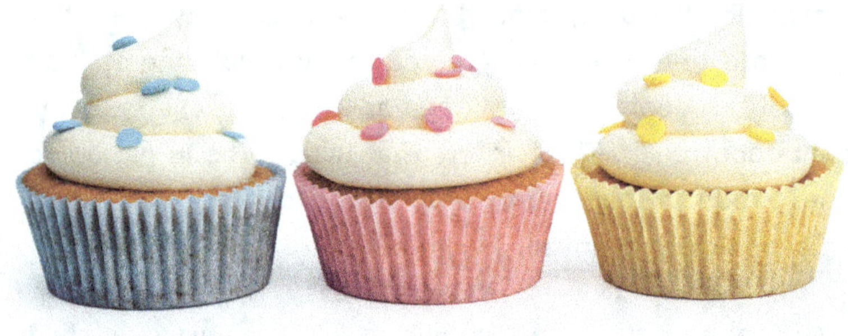

A gluten free diet is one that does not include foods that contain the protein known as gluten. Gluten can be found in wheat, malts, rye, triticale, and barley. It is commonly used as an additive in foods to add more flavors, to thicken foods, to stabilize foods, and is often labeled as "dextrin". A diet free from gluten is the only type of treatment that has been medically accepted for the condition of celiac disease, wheat allergies, and dermatitis herpetiformis.

In some cases, a gluten free diet may not include oats. The medical community is not sure whether or not oats irritate celiac disease patients, or if they cause issues because of cross contamination in processing facilities.

The phrase "gluten free" is used to indicate either a complete lack, or a miniscule amount of gluten. In most cases, gluten free means there is a harmless amount of the protein since a complete absence is unlikely. For the most part, consumption of fewer than

10mg of gluten on a daily basis is unlikely to cause any allergic reactions or problems in gluten sensitive patients.

Starting on a gluten free diet does not have to be difficult, and you do not need to feel deprived. Some basic guidelines can help you through the process.

The first step to switching your way of eating is to focus on foods you know you can have. These include vegetables and fruits, fruit juices, plain milk that has not flavored, unflavored teas, coffee beans, eggs, corn, potatoes, nuts, legumes, beans, oils, and meats and fish that are not coated, breaded, process, or marinated. You can also safely add herbs and spices, since these are quite flavorful and are completely gluten free.

Although the above mentioned grains need to be avoided, there are some grains that are safe, and gluten free. These include: Montina, Rice, Teff, Amaranth, Sorghum, Buckwheat, Quinoa, Corn, and Soy (but not soy sauce that is made from wheat).

There are also a variety of gluten free flours that can be used to make baked goods, food coatings, and other food products. This flour is made from gluten free grains that have been ground into flour, as well as nuts, beans, potatoes, and tapioca.

Today, gluten free flour can easily be found in most supermarkets, as well as health food stores. Since the gluten free lifestyle is growing in popularity, there are also a number of gluten free baking mixes to make cakes, muffins, breads, cookies, and the like, as well as readymade gluten free food products such as bagels, pizza, and tortillas.

Of course, let's not forget about pasta. There is now a variety of gluten free pastas that are sold in many food markets that are made from buckwheat, corn, rice, and quinoa. Noodles are also commonly made from buckwheat and are quite safe for gluten free dieters.

Why Go Gluten Free?

As previously mentioned, there are many a variety of health issues that make it necessary for some people to begin a gluten free diet. For these people, eating bread, or even having a beer can cause severe pain in the abdominal area, bloating, gas, and diarrhea.

In more serious cases, such as for those who suffer with celiac disease, eating foods that contain gluten can trigger a response by the autoimmune system that actually causes damage to the small intestine and prevents proper absorption of certain nutrients.

While these medical issues can be quite serious, and cause severe allergies for some, why on earth would anyone opt for this type of diet and give up all of their favorite foods in their traditional forms if they do not have to?

Many Hollywood stars, personal trainers, and fitness gurus are going the gluten free route, so there must be something to this mysterious diet. This section will explain some of the most common and important reasons to eliminate gluten, as well as other positive benefits for those without allergies.

What is Celiac Disease?

Celiac disease is a type of autoimmune disease that is inherited, and causes damage to the small intestine when gluten and other forms of proteins that is found in wheat, rye, barley, and in some cases, oats, is eaten.

Since symptoms of celiac disease can vary a great deal from patient to patient, a delay in a proper diagnosis is quite common. While many cases of celiac disease go undiagnosed, it is estimated that nearly one in one hundred thirty three people suffer with the condition. In some people, constipation may be the main symptom, while in others diarrhea is, and yet in many others, there is no stool irregularity.

Other common symptoms of celiac disease include:

• Abdominal pain,

• Gas,

• bloating,

• Indigestion,

• A distended stomach,

• Nausea,

• vomiting,

• A decrease in appetite,

• Intolerance to lactose,

• Weight loss that cannot be explained,

• And stools that float, have blood in them, appear fatty, or are quite foul smelling.

Other non digestive related symptoms include:

• bruising easily,

• Pain in the joints or bones,

• Depression,

• Children with growth delays,

• Hair loss,

• Fatigue,

• Malnutrition,

• Changes in behavior,

• Anemia,

• Irritability,

• Skin problems,

• Seizures,

• Ulcers in the mouth,

• Decrease in bone density,

• Muscle cramps,

• swelling,

• Hypoglycemia,

• Nose bleeds,

• Difficulty breathing or catching the breath,

• Defects in tooth enamel or discolorations,

• And deficiencies in vitamins or minerals such as folate, vitamin K, or iron.

CHAPTER 3- GLUTEN FREE MEAL – HEALTHY LIFE

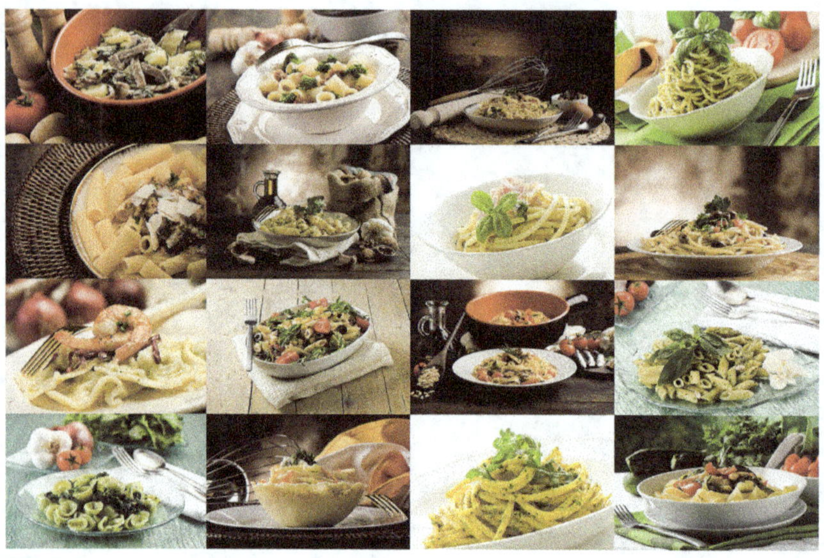

Autism is a disorder that is becoming a major concern amongst parents, pediatricians, and even educators. Because this disorder seems to be becoming more common, it has sparked a great deal of debate and research into the reason behind its development.

New studies, especially those that have been based in the alternative medicine field, have found that there could be a potential link between food allergies and autism, especially a link between gluten and the condition.

This new data suggest that gluten may create allergies that either cause or worsen autism.

Autism is a disorder that affects children's cognitive development and cognitive function. This can cause problems with communication abilities, behavior, and social interaction. While it was thought that autism may be genetic, recent studies have found that environmental factors may actually be cause of, or influence the disorder.

The studies that tracked autism with gluten allergies found that the food proteins in these foods were broken down into small proteins known as peptides. This then functioned as a narcotic would in autistic children, causing outward symptoms to worsen.

Since allergic responses to gluten can affect the body on the whole, causing a variety of mental and physical symptoms, the consequences can be far reaching. "Brain fog" is considered to be a mental symptom of autism, but is also often mistaken for other psychiatric conditions.

Gluten intolerant adults are often plagued by physical symptoms of consuming gluten foods, while children tend to suffer more from mental side effects, such as brain fog.

Just as the remedy for a gluten intolerant adult is a gluten free diet, parents with children showing symptoms of mental impairment may want to consider eliminating gluten in the daily diet. Once parents cut out gluten, mental changes are often reported in a very short period of time. Cognitive problems, abnormal behavior, antisocial tendencies, and problems with communication have completely disappeared in many cases.

Top Ten Reasons to Go Gluten Free

Even if you do not have an intolerance or allergy to gluten, giving up gluten filled foods can do wonders for your health. Below are ten reasons why anyone should consider going gluten free.

If you can get nutrition from gluten, you can get it from other sources as well.

Most gluten filled grains are high in dietary fiber and various types of B vitamins. This is why so many people believe it is so important to eat these foods. What most people do not know is that if you can get this nutrition from gluten based grains, you can get it in other foods.

For example, one hundred grams of whole wheat flour provides thirty percent of the recommended allowance of niacin, and thirty two percent of the recommended allowance of thiamin. Eating sesame seeds or flaxseeds provides even more of these nutrients, while being completely gluten free.

Many foods containing gluten are also touted as being fiber rich. This too is an issue that can easily be remedied with other foods. For example, one hundred grams of brown rice has just less than two grams of fiber. In comparison, collard greens have nearly three grams of fiber, and green peas have nearly five grams of fiber.

Grains containing gluten are not good for your stomach.

When your stomach is not healthy, the rest of your body will not feel healthy because you will not be able to absorb all of the necessary nutrients from food. This in turn makes your body more prone to illness, and even at risk for becoming malnourished. Gluten filled foods have been linked to a condition known as "leaky gut syndrome".

This means that tiny pieces of the foods are leaked out of the intestinal walls causing the body to react with an immune response. When the immune system is taxed in this way it cannot effectively fight of illnesses.

You may be unable to process gluten properly.

Many Caucasian people have a higher risk for being unable to properly digest gluten rich foods. While research has estimated that about one percent of the population has celiac disease, the numbers may actually be quite a bit higher. Some studies have estimated that nearly thirty to forty percent of people of European descent have some form or degree of gluten allergy.

Gluten causes inflammation.

Because these types of grain are high in starch, they tend to be inflammatory. The more refined grains you eat, the more inflammation is possible. Take unbleached white flour for example. This ingredient is much more inflammatory than even whole wheat flour.

That being said, foods that are gluten free such as fresh vegetables and healthy fats have been shown to reduce inflammation. People who suffer with chronic inflammation have been subjected to many different conditions such as allergies, bone loss, arthritis, asthma, cardiovascular disease, and even some types of cancer.

Gluten grains are fairly new types of food.

Even though grains containing gluten are considered to be whole foods, and nutritious, they are still relatively new to the human diet. Before the birth of agriculture, human beings simply hunted and gathered their foods. This meant eating animal protein, fish, wild berries, fruits, wild greens, nuts, and the like. Our ancestors did not plant gardens, they did not harvest grains, and they did not drink dairy products.

Humans survived on this diet for a great many years, before grains ever became introduced. Today, grains now account for the bulk of our modern diet, which has led to a variety of new health conditions.

Gluten grains can harm your joints.

As previously explained, gluten filled grains are quite inflammatory. This also wreaks havoc on your joints, leading to painful conditions such as arthritis. These types of foods contain amino acids that mimic those already found in the joints' soft tissues.

Since both components are quite similar in makeup, the body has great difficulty telling which is natural and which is introduced. This leads to cells becoming overworked, and inflamed, which triggers the immune system to fight off foreign bodies. Unfortunately the immune system really ends up attacking the joints themselves.

Gluten grains can block minerals from being properly absorbed.

When gluten grains are not prepared properly, and in most cases today they are not, they can actually prevent vitamins and minerals from being absorbed into the body.

Even though you may be eating a diet that has plenty of calcium, iron, and other important nutrients, if you eat gluten filled grains that are not prepared correctly, you will not be able to absorb all of the foods nutrients.

The only exception to this is to sprout certain grains and eat the sprouts as this makes the grains more absorbable by the body.

Gluten grains can harm your teeth.

Grains that contain gluten have high phytate levels, which have been attributed to tooth decay. Pytates, or phytic acid, has been shown to block mineral absorption causing bacteria to feed on the starches leading to tooth decay.

Gluten grains are not good for the skin.

Glutens tend to be found in foods that are very high in carbohydrates, and while not all carbohydrates are bad, they are broken down into various types of sugars. Sugar tells the body to produce insulin, which can in turn trigger hormonal responses that cause the sebum producing glands in the skin to produce more oil. This can contribute to acne, and other skin related conditions.

Consuming gluten makes your body crave gluten.

Just about everyone has had the experience of smelling a freshly baked loaf of bread and all of a sudden craving a nice thick, warm slice. How about freshly baked cookies? A nice warm, gooey plate in front of you makes it nearly impossible to eat just one. Foods that are high in carbohydrates provide a quick burst of energy.

However, that burst of energy wears off quickly, and then the body is left wanting more. This causes a rise and fall in insulin levels, which can lead to more and more gluten being craved, so the cycle continues.

CHAPTER 4- GLUTEN FREE DIET EVERYDAY

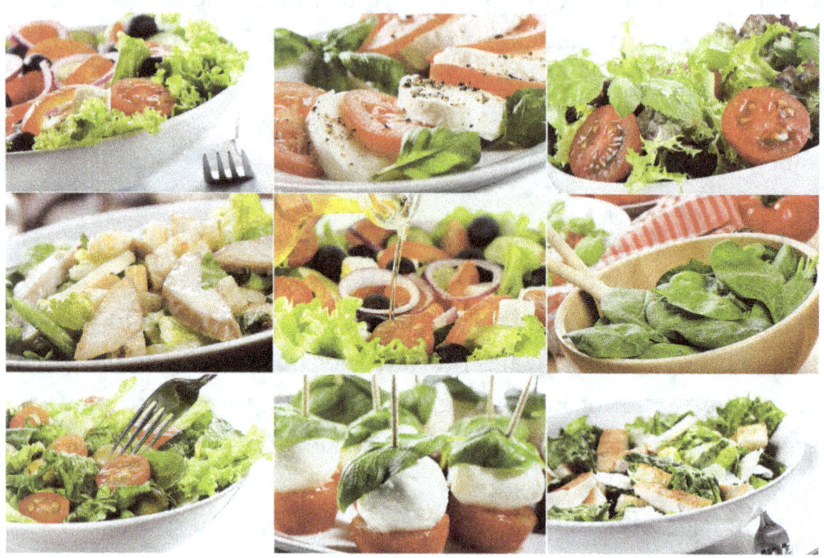

Just as with any type of diet, a gluten free diet can be as healthy or unhealthy as you make it. That being said, you should be aware of how to make the best choices to get the very most out of your gluten free diet.

Multivitamins

A good multivitamin can be a great idea, no matter what type of diet you eat. This can help bridge any nutritional gaps in your diet, and keep you as healthy as possible. If you are not sure what type of multivitamin is best for your needs, contact your doctor or pharmacist for more information.

These professionals should be able to recommend a good option to meet your specific needs.

Constipation

The types of grains that are considered to be safe for a gluten free diet are often somewhat low in fiber. This is particularly true for rice, and rice based products. If you eat a fair amount of these foods, you body may not be getting enough fiber. To help with this issue, you can eat more fresh fruits and vegetables, which should help with constipation. You may also need an over the counter solution in some cases; just verify it is gluten free before use.

Stay Away from Junk Food

Just because cookies, cakes, breads, and brownies advertise themselves as being gluten free, does not mean they are completely healthy. You should be just as wary of these foods as you would if they contained gluten.

Having dessert occasionally is fine. Eating sweets daily is probably not a good idea.

Think Low Carb

This does not mean that you have to go "carb crazy" and cut them out entirely. However, sticking to a lower carb diet can be beneficial, when you eat plenty of fresh fruits and vegetables, and lean sources of protein.

Exercise

Just as with other types of diets, a good exercise program can do wonders for your health, even when on a gluten free diet. Studies show that even just thirty minutes of brisk exercise per day can be quite beneficial. A simple walk down the street, a short jog, or a play session in the back yard with your kids can raise your heart rate, burn extra calories, and make you feel better all the way around.

Staying healthy without gluten does not have to be a big mystery. The same concepts you would incorporate into your life if you were not gluten free, essentially hold true when you are. Remember to limit refined foods, watch your junk intake, increase the amount of fruits and vegetables you eat, and get plenty of exercise. It is just that simple.

Transforming Your Pantry to be Gluten Free

One area many people who decide to go gluten free struggle with is transforming the pantry to be rid of foods they can no longer eat. As tedious as it may sound, the best way to begin the process is to take the list of ingredients that contain gluten, and read every food item's label in your kitchen.

Of course there are obvious foods such as cereal, bread, pasta, and processed items that need to be tossed. You should also check certain mixes and rice dishes as they often contain wheat thickeners.

Once you have finished with the obvious items, it is then time to check on the less obvious items. Spice blends, mixed salts, and even vanilla extract need to go. Soy sauce, condiments, and salad dressings next to be checked for problematic additives, canned soups should be checked because they often use wheat thickeners, and soup starters, broths, bouillons, and gravy mixes should all be examined.

Next, check frozen food dinners, vegetables in sauces, and prepared dishes that often list gluten on the package. If you cannot verify the ingredients, you may want to err on the side of caution and toss the item.

From this point, you will need to decide what type of pantry you want to have. Do you want to have an entirely gluten free pantry for everyone in the family? This will mean that even those members of your family who can eat gluten will only eat gluten free foods.

If you are not sure this is the way you want to proceed, you may opt for a combined pantry. This means that there will be a separation of food items that contain gluten and those that do not, and it will be clearly set up to avoid confusion. While this may seem like the perfect compromise, you should be aware that there is always the potential that foods will be cross contaminated if the same utensils are used for serving, or containers are mixed up.

Should you opt to go completely gluten free, you should consider donating any unopened food items and canned goods to a local soup kitchen or food pantry. You may also want to see if your friends or coworkers could use the miscellaneous items such as frozen foods or spices.

Shopping Tips

The grocery store can be an intimidating place for a person who is gluten free. In order to get the most out of your shopping trip, yet ensure your food choices are completely safe, it is best to approach the store by sections.

Let's begin by taking a virtual trip around the grocery store to highlight the safest areas for gluten free shoppers.

The first stop in most grocery stores is the produce section. This section is completely safe, so you should spend a good amount of time here. Make sure you choose a variety of fresh produce, with a range of colors. Choose deep leafy greens, oranges, reds, and even purples for your diet.

The next stop is the meat section. Since meat, poultry, and fish are excellent sources of vitamins, minerals, good fats, and protein, you should be sure to choose a nice selection of items. The only items you need to steer clear of are those that are prepared, pre-coated, or marinated. You can even choose deli meats, as long as they are just plain meat, or plain cheese products.

From here it is time to move on to the dairy section. Most items found in this department are considered to be safe. Milk, yogurt, eggs, butter, and cheese are all acceptable foods. You should opt for skim milk or whole milk products, over fat free items. Fat free foods can contain additives to make the product appear thicker, so avoiding these foods is a safe bet.

As you navigate your way around the perimeter of the store you will find the bakery is usually the next stop. Just keep on walking, since most products here are off limits!

Once you have made all of the above mentioned safe and healthy choices, you can then move on to the interior aisles of the store.

The frozen food section can be a bit daunting. Here you should stick to plain fruits, vegetables, and meat items. Stay away from products with sauces, seasonings, or coatings.

The dried and canned food aisles are safe for the most part. Again, stick to plain foods, with no extra ingredients. Dried beans are cheap and nutritious, and are packed with minerals, vitamins, and protein. Canned vegetable, fruits, beans, and juices are all safe for the most part and provide a good amount of flavor. Canned soups should be avoided as they are often thickened with wheat.

That's it! That is all of the aisles you should be visiting while sticking to a gluten free diet. If you stick to this outline and some basic guidelines you will have successfully navigated your way through the grocery store with ease. In time, you will find it will become second nature to select food items that are both safe and nutritious.

Focus on Your Meals

Planning your meals is an important part of a gluten free lifestyle. It reduces the need for you to make an unhealthy choice because you are pushed for time. Plan your snacks too so that you always have something you can reach for when you get hungry. You don't have to be overwhelmed by the task of going to the grocery store though.

There are more stores that offer gluten free products than you may realize. The demand for them as well as the variety of options continues to grow all the time. You can go online to find out where to shop locally for those items you want. If you aren't finding enough selection, talk to the manager.

They may be willing to add a few gluten free items to what they normally stock if customers ask for it. Studies show that as of 2012, approximately 15% of customers were shopping for only gluten free products. Up to 25% were buying products gluten free as they have scaled down on the volume of gluten that they consume.

The predictions from U.S. News and World Report are that this percentage is only going to continue to climb in the future.

Retailers that sell groceries are certainly going to be paying attention to this information as well and preparing the shelves in their stores to meet that demand.

Being well informed is important when you are shopping for gluten free products. Some of the common foods you may normally reach for to add to your basket contain gluten including:

• Bagels

• Cereal

• Crackers

• Pasta

• Pizza

Identifying what you can safely eat and what you can't is important so that you can be a great shopper. To help you feel better about all of this, focus on what you can eat and not what you are giving up.

Remember the many health benefits that you will gain when you start to feel your willpower slipping. The more you shop for gluten free items, the easier it becomes. Soon, it will be second nature for you when you enter the store.

Carefully Read Labels!

Different brands of products can contain gluten or not so you need to become familiar with the products out there. Don't be in a rush when you shop so that you can take all the time you need to read labels. Some products say gluten free and others say low gluten.

Fruits and Vegetables

Any fresh fruits and fresh vegetables that you see in the grocery store aren't processed and they are gluten free. You can buy sweet potatoes and white potatoes as they don't contain any gluten either. Both dry beans and peas are acceptable.

Dairy

Just about all of the milk and cheese that you will find at the grocery store are free of gluten. There are some exceptions though so you need to carefully read labels. Some processed cheese products have wheat in them and blue cheese does. If you buy plain yogurt there is no gluten. However, if you buy various flavors then there can be so always check the labels.

Meat, Fish, Pork, & Poultry

Look for lean cuts of meat, pork, and poultry. Only buy fresh fish and other forms of seafood. When you are looking at canned or frozen products in this category, many of them can contain gluten due to the processing. Always take the time to carefully read the labels. When possible, use fresh products instead of frozen or canned as they are better for you.

Grains

Select grains that are free of gluten. You will find that you can pick the varieties you like too. There are gluten free options with white, brown, and wild rice so your choice won't be limited.

When it comes to dining out, spend some time looking online to identify which restaurants offer you such dishes. This is very important if you are traveling and aren't familiar with the area. With the technology today, you can use your Smartphone or a laptop to see what is available where you happen to be.

If you aren't able to do that, ask when you arrive about any gluten free foods that they may offer. Some locations are willing to make something special for you. With more restaurants trying to appease the needs of everyone it is possible they will work with you. Try to arrive at off peak times so they can provide you with personalized service.

There are some common items you can get though that would be fine. For example, order chicken or fish with a side of vegetables. You can also get a baked potato and a salad. You may want to ask what type of oil that fish or chicken is cooked in though as some of them do contain gluten.

There is a great deal of gluten in various marinades and sauces. If you aren't sure they are free of gluten it is best to avoid them. You can ask for them to be put on the side and most restaurants will be happy to comply.

Don't expect there to be gluten free bread or crackers though so make sure you don't reach for them unless you are positive!

It is fine to consume champagne and wine as they are made from grapes. However, most beer is going to be off limits due to the grains they use to make them. You will find some gluten free beer offers though in many restaurants so it doesn't hurt to ask. You can also consider various forms of mixed drinks.

If dessert is something you just don't want to pass up, you aren't going to have to. There are some great choices in this category too. If the restaurant is gluten free friendly they may have flourless cake available. You can also consider sorbet, sherbet, fresh fruit, or ice cream. They are universal options so there is a very good chance they will be available.

Some labels on products aren't as clear as they should be when it comes to determining if they contain gluten or not. If that is the case with a particular product, err on the side of caution. Don't buy it and you can do some research at home about it. You can always buy that product on your next shopping trip if you do find it is actually free of gluten.

The more you are aware of what you can eat and what you shouldn't, the easier it is for you to shop and for your to dine out without stress or worry. See appendix 1 for a list to help you as you work to become more familiar with your options.

Meal Prep Tips

Much the same as other diet plans, a good gluten free diet begins each day with breakfast. Breakfast is the most important meal of the day, and can provide a wide range of health benefits. When you are eating a gluten free diet, breakfast can also help to keep your appetite even throughout the day, making it easier to avoid craving gluten free foods.

You should always opt to keep a range of breakfast items on hand at all times, so it is never a struggle to put together a nutritious morning meal. Gluten free cereals, gluten free waffles, gluten free muffins, fresh fruit, frozen fruit, dried fruit, eggs, and gluten free cereal bars are all great options.

Once you have conquered breakfast, you need to devise a plan for lunch. Because of hectic schedules, it is not always easy to slow down and take time for the perfect lunch. By packing your lunch you will be able to know you are eating safely, eating well, saving time, and even saving money.

Why is Gluten Free Living a Good Idea?

Some individuals have no choice but to follow a gluten free lifestyle due to the way their bodies process it. Celiac disease is a type of autoimmune disorder that results in the body rejecting gluten instead of processing it. The gluten is seen as a toxin to their bodies and it can create very serious health problems.

The severity of the reaction can vary based on the individual and the amount of gluten that they consume. A gluten allergy is extremely common, but it is very rarely diagnosed. Today, more people are informed about the symptoms and more medical professionals are testing for it.

This is why the number of children with sensitivity to gluten is being identified. There are adults that have struggled with their health for their entire life though because this gluten problem was never addressed. The sooner that a person is diagnosed though the sooner changes to their diet can be implemented.

It is believed that 1 in 133 people have some form of Celiac disease. The problem is that when they are consuming gluten their small intestine is being damaged. This creates problems with the small intestine successfully absorbing nutrients that the body needs. Some reports indicate approximately 83% of the cases though aren't diagnosed.

Children may have some other symptoms that develop including:

• Behavioral changes

• Dental enamel damage

• Distended abdomen

• Failure to gain weight or height at their percentile

In order to confirm such a diagnosis, blood work is completed. If it comes back positive, than a biopsy of the small intestine will be done to see if the lining has been damaged as well as the degree of any damage that has occurred. There is no cure for Celiac disease other than to follow a gluten free diet.

Doing so allow the small intestine to heal and in time it can allow a person to make a full recovery. Their body will start being able to use the nutrients that they consume for better overall health. The problem will get worse if dietary changes aren't made including malnutrition, osteoporosis, neurological problems, and Lymphoma.

If possible, request for a test for you and your children. This is because so many people go undiagnosed with this type of problem. If you think this could be the issue, don't want until your doctor brings up the idea of the testing. Ask your family members too in order to determine if there is a high chance of it occurring for you or your child.

Some individuals develop Dermatitis Herpetiformis, often referred to as DH, which is a type of Celiac disease that affects the skin. In order to diagnosis it blood work and a skin biopsy are conducted. The only cure for it is also a gluten free diet.

Such a test is a good idea as this type of skin problem is often mistaken for Eczema. It can be very frustrating when the medication for Eczema is given but the condition either stays the same or gets worse. Until the diet is changed then the skin isn't going to clear up.

Many people make the choice to have a gluten free diet even though they don't have the disease. Some have a family history of many health problems and they are being as proactive as possible to reduce the risk of serious health concerns for them personally.

If you decide to make this your lifestyle due to your own personal beliefs, you need to stand up for it. Don't let others that don't agree with you or that don't understand your decision to create problems or doubts for you. Not everyone in your life will be supportive about it but the majority of people will.

A gluten free lifestyle isn't something to be shy about, to be ashamed of, or that you need to hide. It may be different from other people and the food choices they make but that is okay. It is about doing what is right for you and for your family in this regard so don't succumb to peer pressure.

Parents try to do all they can to create a world for their children that is fair, that is fun, and that is rewarding. Yet there can be issues with children that society as a whole isn't kind about, for example, children that have ADD or ADHD or those with Autism.

As the parent of a child with those types of issues, it can be exhausting. It can be hard for you and your partner to deal with on a daily basis. You may feel like you have been isolated by your friends and family because of it. Not giving up on your child though is important.

Some parents have found that their child did significantly improve by removing gluten from their diet. This was a better option for them than medicating their child. When there are behavior issues that aren't explained, it is definitely worth trying a gluten free diet for a few months and monitoring the behavior of your child.

If you see improvements, then that is encouraging and you should continue the diet. It could make a huge difference in the happiness of your child, in the dynamics of your household, and even how your child is accepted socially.

There are a few studies out there that indicate a gluten free diet can be a way to reduce symptoms of other forms of autoimmune deficiencies too. This includes:

• Cystic Fibrosis

• Multiple Sclerosis

• Thyroid Disease

Such information is very encouraging because it can be very upsetting to deal with the symptoms of these autoimmune deficiencies. They can create pain, fatigue, and other symptoms that affect every element of a person's life. If changing to a gluten free diet can make these health problems more manageable, isn't it worth it to consider?

Other individuals have taken on a gluten free lifestyle due to having a child or partner that needs to follow such a diet plan. It is certainly easier to create meals that everyone in the household can consume rather than making something different from the person that can't have gluten. Plus, if a parent has gluten related issue that it is very possible children in the household will at some point.

Teaching them a healthier way of eating from an early age is important.

There are people that choose not to consume gluten because they feel better removing it from their diet. While they didn't test positive for Celiac disease, they may have some sort of wheat allergy. They may have an intolerance or sensitivity to gluten.

They often have gas or bloating when they consume it so they have removed if from their diet to be more comfortable. They don't have damage to the small intestine due to the gluten but they just feel better overall by not consuming it anymore.

No one wants to try to get through their day continually with bloating and gas. It can make it hard to focus on work, social activities, and even intimate relationships. With the anxiety gone about such symptoms, it can give a person a refreshing and upbeat outlook about life that was missing before.

Weight loss and weight maintenance has also been a reason to stop consuming gluten. The craving for sweets can make it hard to stick to a good diet plan but many people find they don't have cravings after a few weeks of a gluten free diet.

They also find that they lose weight and keep it off because they are no longer reaching for foods that have empty calories or snacks that are processed. Such changes can also do wonders for the amount of energy a person has.

Many people feel that they have been on a losing course for weight loss for quite some time. They don't have the willpower to stick with a program that is restricting them and they really shouldn't. Fad diets may be very popular but they are really just setting people up to fail. Many people find that they can stick with a gluten free diet and that they do lose weight.

There are a few reasons for that to occur. As previously mentioned, the cravings go away and that makes selecting healthier choices easier. Reducing the amount of processed foods that are consumed means that there is less harmful carbs that the body will store as fat. There is also less sugar intake that will be stored as fat.

The increased energy with this lifestyle also gives someone that help them may need to really exercise. They may have had a hard time doing so before but now they have both the energy and the motivation to stick with a plan of action. As they feel better and their mood improves it becomes a path that they would like to continue going down.

The verdict is still out there by the experts though regarding recommending the gluten free diet for weight loss. Since it can't be proven without in depth and time consuming studies you won't find doctor's that readily recommend it. However, you will find plenty of people that state it was the change that allowed them to feel great and to drop the pounds when nothing else worked.

If you have hit a point where you feel like losing weight is a lost cause, you may wish to give this type of lifestyle a try for a 90 day period. If you find that you feel better, you have more energy, and that you have lost weight then it is an option to continue with it.

Regardless of your reason for deciding to follow a gluten free diet – by necessity or by choice – it doesn't have to be hard and it doesn't have to be time consuming. It doesn't mean that you have a huge grocery bill or that you can't enjoy going out to eat.

If you travel often, you may be worried but you can use the internet to help you find great menu choices and restaurants anywhere you may go that offer gluten free selections. You have the ability to make this work for you and all of the information you need is at your fingertips!

A thermos of gluten free soup, fresh fruit and yogurt, leftovers from dinner the night before, and vegetables with hummus are delicious lunch options. Since most of us love our snacks, you should plan to have some snacking options to keep your hunger under control. Snacks should be no more than one hundred to two hundred calories, and can be items such as rice crackers with peanut butter, fruit, cheese cubes, or gluten free protein bar.

Dinner will most likely be your largest and most elaborate meal of the day. The majority of your meal should consist of freshly cooked veggies, or a nice big salad, a lean protein source, and a nice side dish such as steamed wild rice, or some beans.

Of course you can experiment as much or as little as you like, but you should try to incorporate variety to keep boredom from setting in. As long as you make your own meals with gluten free ingredients that you have stocked in your gluten free pantry you will find you look better, feel better, and can be proud you are doing something healthy for yourself and your family.

Gluten Free Snacks and Sweets

You certainly do not have to give up all of your favorite snacks and sweets just because you have decided to go gluten free. Because so many people have decided to give up gluten and get healthy, there are more products than ever on the market that are safe, and delicious.

Today, there is a full range of gluten free chips, crackers, cookies, cakes, brownies, and even candy bars. These premade convenience foods can be great for people on the go, for packing in lunches, and to help ward off those pesky cravings.

Chapter 5- Gluten Problem – What to do?

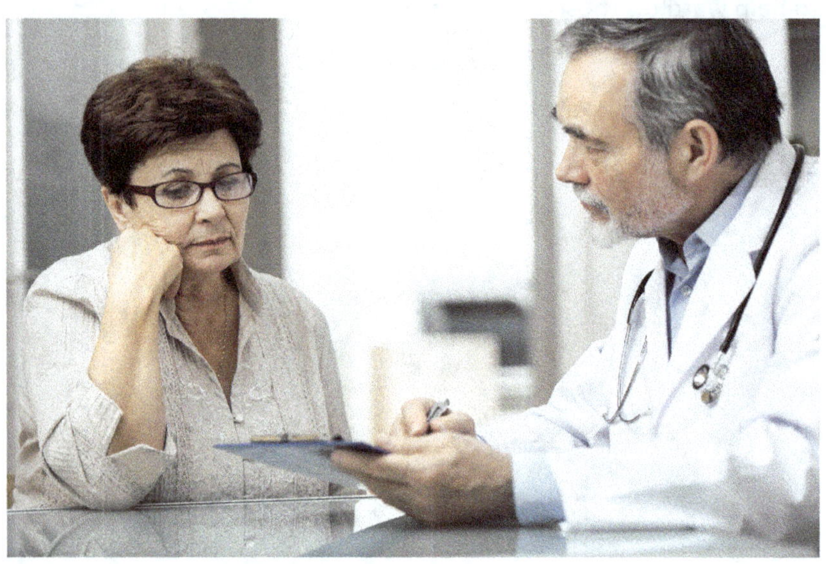

See your Doctor

It isn't recommended to self diagnose when it comes to a gluten problem. You should consult with your doctor to have the correct testing done. Some of the symptoms of gluten problems can be the same as other forms of health problems so it is important to get a professional diagnosis.

Continue to eat the way you normally would though when you are scheduled for the testing. If there is no gluten in your body then the blood work isn't going to be able to determine that it is the core of the problem (if indeed it is)! If your blood work shows that there is a problem then you can remove the gluten.

Of course if you are making the change because you want to and not because of a medical concern then you can make the change when you are ready. Either use up the items you have in your home with gluten or toss them out and make a fresh break from it.

Many people find tossing those items in the trash is quite empowering!

The outreach in place for this type of testing has significantly grown in the past couple of years. Part of the education process involves getting more doctors to prescribe such testing for their patients. By 2019 the goal is to successfully diagnose as many cases as possible so that children and adults with a gluten concern aren't slipping through the cracks and increasing the risk of serious health problems.

Some individuals will still notice they have some symptoms even after they switch to a gluten free diet. This can be due to the severity of their condition. It can also be due to the damage that has occurred for the small intestine. While the small intestine is healing itself, your doctor may recommend that you take dietary supplements in order if malnourishment has occurred.

Many individuals that are changing to a gluten free diet aren't getting the amount of certain vitamins that their body needs. Your doctor may recommend a supplement to increase the amount of Vitamin B, iron, zinc, or calcium. If such supplements are recommended take them until your doctor feels you no longer need them.

Household Items to Watch for

Most people have the understanding that gluten is only found in foods that you consume. However, there are some household items that may contain it so you need to be diligent in looking at them too. Here are the most common ones that you need to take a very close look at before you use them again.

It will depend on the brand so you need to read the label:

• Chapstick

• Glue

• Gum

• Medicines (Including over the counter, herbal remedies, and prescriptions)

• Toothpaste

CHAPTER 6- GLUTEN FREE RECIPES

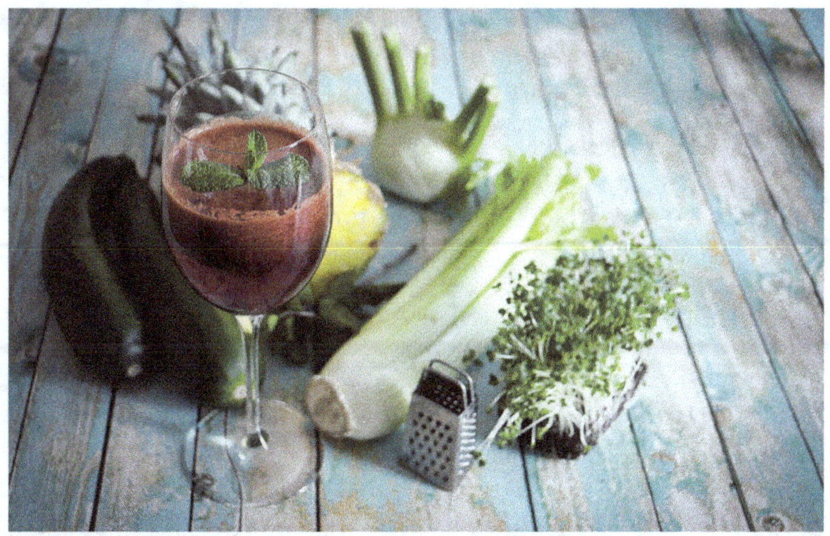

It is a good idea to add the following items to your shopping list and to keep them on hand in your kitchen. They are commonly called for in gluten free recipes. You can also use them when you run low on food items for your menu to make something.

• Gluten free baking mix

• Gluten free crackers

• Gluten free bread crumbs

• Gluten free flour

• Gluten free snacks

• Guar Gum

• Quinoa

• Rice (brown or white depending on your preference)

• Xantham Gum

With these items you can also use some of your favorite recipes but with a gluten free value to them. It can be both fun and productive to get creative with those recipes. Here are some great tips for starting with such replacements:

• Binders – Use Xanthan Gum, Guar Gum, or gelatin.

• Breading – Wheat or gluten free bread crumbs or crushed potato chips.

• Flour – Use gluten free flour mix or cornstarch. There are plenty of options to consider including amaranth and sorghum.

• Thickening – Use cornstarch or gluten free baking mix. For a sweet recipe, use dry pudding mix.

The internet is a wonderful resource for finding various gluten free recipes to try. You will enjoy the new tastes and you will gain more confidence in this lifestyle choice as you are able to create meals you and your family love.

You can also buy gluten free cookbooks, magazines, or exchange recipes with others that are also eating gluten free.

Here are some great ideas to get you started. Try some new recipes and create a file for those that you really like.

As your file grows you can ensure lots of variety in your diet so you don't feel restricted or bored by eating the same thing over and over again.

Breakfast Ideas

Yogurt is a great option but make sure it is gluten free as many varieties aren't. Both Stonyfield and Chobani are certified by the Gluten Intolerant Group. You can use the yogurt as a basis for a delicious tasting smoothie too.

There are various brands of gluten free cereal by General Mills and Nature's Path. If you like hot cereal, consider Cream of Buckwheat. There are also oats that are certified to be gluten free. Eggs that are fried or scrambled are a great way to start the day due to the amount of protein they offer.

Lunch Ideas

Lunch meat is a great choice for a convenient and gluten free option, but make sure it isn't processed. A salad can be a choice that works for you due to all of the vegetables. You have to be careful though as some of the cheese items and various dressings can have gluten in them.

Nachos consisting of tortilla chips and some melted cheese that is gluten free is a change from your basic lunch and very appetizing. Peanut butter on gluten free bread is another great consideration.

Dinner Ideas

Lean cuts of meat including beef, pork, and poultry are great choices. You can also consume fresh fish or other seafood. Adding fresh vegetables and your choice of potatoes offers you a wonderful meal without gluten in no time at all. You can also replace the potatoes with your choice of gluten free rice.

Snack Ideas

Gluten free snacks you can enjoy between meals will keep you on track. Cut up fresh fruit and vegetables so you can grab them and go. You can pack them to take in the car or to have at your desk while working.

There are plenty of types of cheese that don't contain gluten, and they are wonderful for snacking. They also help you to get your calcium. With certain flavors of cheese you need to be careful as they can have some gluten in them so always read the packaging. Kids seem to really enjoy those individually wrapped cheese sticks.

While you should only consume chips in moderation, they are also gluten free when it comes to many varieties including most of those offered by Frito Lay. For a lower calorie snack consider popcorn. Make some hardboiled eggs and consume them when you need a snack. They will give you lots of energy.

Dessert Ideas

Both children and adults enjoy dessert, and you don't have to eliminate it due to a gluten free diet. Various brands of pudding are free of gluten and you will have a variety of flavors to pick from. Ice cream can also be a wonderful treat but you need to pay attention to the labels. So many ice cream varieties these days are packed with goodies so you need to pay attention to what is in there.

Cross Contamination

It is very important that you think about the risk of cross contamination in your own kitchen as well as those of others that prepare gluten free meals for you or your family. If the same tools are used to prepare such items as those that do have gluten then there can be some contamination.

Even a small amount of gluten can be dangerous to certain individuals so care has to be taken to prevent this. It is one more reason why changing the entire family to a gluten free diet may be the best option to consider.

Holidays

For many people, the holidays can be tough due to the restrictions of the diet. There can be parties to attend and various events where you have to be very careful about what you eat.

You may decide to make dinner at your own home and offer a gluten free meal for all. It is certainly an option to consider. Prepare yourself for the holidays and have a few items you can take along for snacks with you in case an event isn't gluten free friendly.

Gluten Free Caramel Corn

5 quarts freshly popped popcorn 2 cups brown sugar

1 cup butter (2 sticks) 1/2 cup light corn syrup 1 teaspoon baking soda

1/4 teaspoon cream of tartar Preheat oven to 250 degrees.

Place the popped popcorn in a large roasting pan. Place butter, sugar, corn syrup, and cream of tartar in a large pan. Heat over medium heat, until melted, stirring often to prevent burning. Bring the mixture to a boil and cook for five minutes longer, stirring continually. Remove from heat. Add baking soda and stir to mix.

Carefully pour the mixture over the popcorn, and stir gently to coat. Bake the entire mixture for 1 hour, stirring every 15 minutes. Remove from the oven and pour onto a large baking sheet to cool. Break up large clumps, and enjoy!

Gluten Free Granola Bars

1 1/2 cups Gluten Free All Purpose Baking Flour 2 cups Gluten Free Rolled Oats

1/4 cup Brown Rice Farina 1 cup Apple Juice

2/3 cup Brown Sugar

2/3 cup Applesauce, unsweetened 1/2 tsp Sea Salt

1/2 tsp Cinnamon, ground 1/4 cup Canola Oil

1 tsp Vanilla 1/2 cup Pecans

3/4 cup Chocolate Chips

Spray a 9 x 13-inch pan with cooking spray. In a large bowl, stir together the flour, oats, farina, cinnamon and salt. Add the brown sugar with a fork. In a separate smaller bowl stir together the apple juice, applesauce, vanilla, and canola oil. Add the wet ingredients to the large bowl with the dry ingredients and blend well.

Stir in the pecans and the chocolate chips and pecans. Spread the mixture into the oiled pan and flatten with a spoon.

Bake at 375°F for 30 minutes. When done, cut into 24 bars and place on two baking trays, ensuring a bit of space between the bars. Place bars back into the oven and bake an additional 10 minutes. Cool on a wire rack.

Some of the Best Gluten Free Dessert Recipes

Gluten Free Chocolate Cake

5 large eggs

8 oz unsweetened chocolate 4 oz semisweet chocolate 1 1/3 cups sugar, divided

1 cup (2 sticks) margarine 1/2 cup water

Preheat oven to 350 degrees.

Lightly coat a 9-inch spring form pan with nonstick cooking spray. Crack the eggs into a small glass or metal bowl and temper them over low heat on the stove, but do not cook. This will allow the eggs to triple in volume when beaten.

In a medium pan, melt the chocolate, water, 1 cup sugar, and margarine over medium heat, stirring continually. Remove from heat and let cool. Transfer the eggs to a mixing bowl. Add the remaining 1/3 cup sugar to the eggs and beat until tripled in volume. Fold the chocolate mixture. Pour the mixture into the prepared pan and bake 30-35 minutes; it will be a little loose in center. Serve warm or room temperature.

Gluten Free Brownies

1 cup gluten free flour

2/3 cup unsweetened cocoa 1/2 teaspoon baking powder

1/3 cup butter or margarine (melted) 1/2 teaspoon salt

1/2 cup brown sugar, packed 1/2 cup granulated sugar

1 large egg

1/3 cup hot water or brewed coffee 1/4 cup chopped walnuts (optional)

Preheat oven to 350 degrees F.

Grease or spray with cooking spray an 8 inch square nonstick pan. Stir together gluten free flour, cocoa, baking powder, and salt. Set aside.

In large mixing bowl, beat butter, sugars, and the egg with an electric mixer on medium speed until well combined. With mixer on low speed, add the dry ingredients, along with the hot water or coffee. Blend well; mixture will be somewhat thick. Stir in walnuts, if desired. Spread batter in prepared pan and bake 20 minutes. Cool the brownies on a wire rack before cutting.

Keeping Kids Happy Around Their Gluten Eating Friends

Children are often the most difficult people to manage when it comes to maintaining a gluten free diet. This is because they like to go out with their friends, go to pizza parties, go to the movies, and all the while do not want to constantly worry about eating foods that may have gluten. When told they cannot have them at all, they feel completely isolated from their gluten eating friends.

So how can you keep kids happy around their friends, but still maintain a gluten free lifestyle?

The main key is to plan ahead. When your child is going to a birthday party, bring a few gluten free cupcakes so he or she can eat a sweet treat with the rest of the kids.

If going out to a pizza restaurant, call ahead and find out if they offer gluten free options, and order a special pizza just for your child. When the child goes to a friend's house for a sleepover, pack a backpack for him or her that is loaded with gluten free chips, gluten free cookies, gluten free brownies, and other fun snacks. This will allow for the full friend experience while still maintaining a safe and healthy lifestyle.

Eating Out While Staying Gluten Free

Just as your child may feel a bit out of place or deprived when going out with his or her friends, you too may feel a bit awkward when going out to dinner with a group of friends or colleagues. Luckily, this issue is much easier to deal with today than in years past.

The first thing that you should do is check with the restaurant in advance to find out if they offer gluten free menu options. More and more local restaurant and even large chains do offer these options.

Be sure to be polite, courteous, and friendly with the wait staff. Take your time and clearly explain your dietary needs, and what you would like; most of the time it is no problem at all.

Make sure you choose options on the menu that are sensible. Choose straightforward foods that you know all of the ingredients. Stay away from dishes with sauces and marinades. When ordering dessert, opt for sherbet, sorbet, ice cream, or a fresh fruit platter.

Eating out while maintaining a gluten free lifestyle does not have to be torture; with a little bit of planning and preparation, you will be able to dine with everyone else without a bit of trouble.

CHAPTER 7- SUPPORT AND PROMOTE GLUTEN FREE DIET

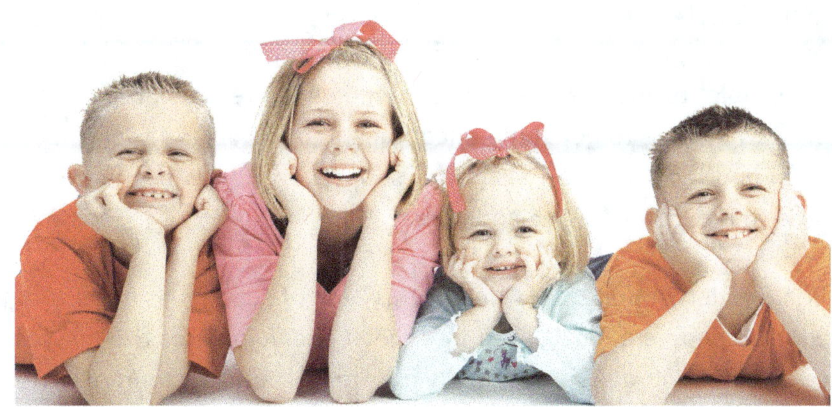

Your decision to be gluten free is one you should feel proud of no matter why you have made that decision. It is a good idea to get a support system in place as soon as you can about it. Share with your family, friends, and co-workers about your lifestyle change and what it entails. You will be pleasantly surprised at the many people that support you and even think about making the change for their own household.

Tell your healthcare providers about such changes too if they haven't mandated it due to a medical necessity. You will find that most medical professionals are very supportive of this type of dietary change.

Being well informed is important so you should consider magazines, books, and websites. However, you need to make sure you fully explore the credibility of such resources or you will end up with so much conflicting information it can make your head spin.

If you have questions, there are some very good organizations where you can direct your questions. They include the Celiac Disease Foundation and the Gluten Intolerance Group.

There are plenty of online forums where you can get support and meet new people. You may find it useful to be able to ask questions from those that are also going through similar changes in their lifestyle.

Being able to share recipes, to vent when you are discouraged, and even to be able to get some encouragement when you really need it is important. You can also offer support to others from time to time so it becomes a give and take.

Don't underestimate the value of this type of support as it helps to educate people about gluten free diets. The volume of the masses can also encourage more gluten free products in restaurants and grocery stores.

If you have children, make sure that their caregivers and teachers know they are on a gluten free diet. You may need to send your child with their lunch daily as the school or daycare lunch menu may not reflect this choice.

You may need to provide snacks too but if you feel this is the right method for your household then your caregiver and the school should work with you. Check to see if there are any gluten free cooking classes offered in your community.

This can be a great way to learn some new cooking methods, try some delicious recipes, and make some terrific friends that you can count on to help you as you help them get used to these dietary changes. You may find working with a dietician is useful as well.

Chapter 8- Gluten Free Take-away

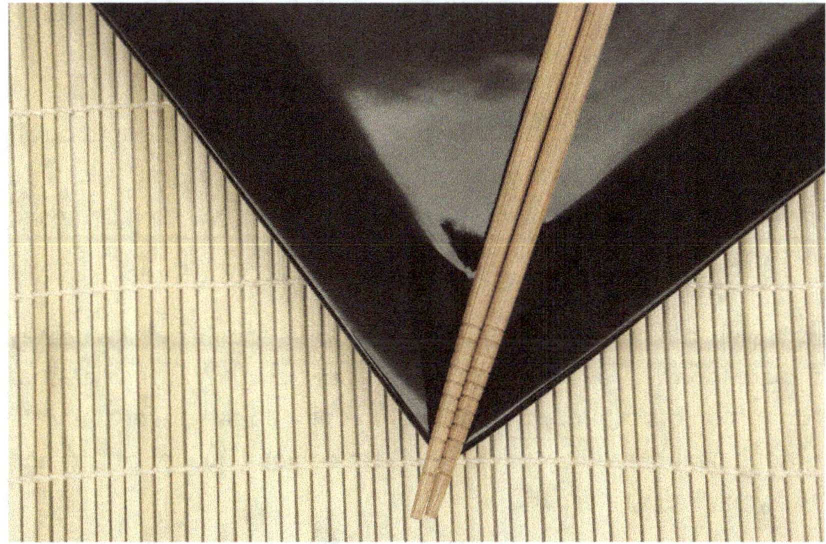

Depending on what you currently eat, changing to a gluten free lifestyle may be a moderate change or a significant change. With the right information, you can accept those changes and become well aware of what you can eat and what you need to steer clear of.

For many individuals, they find that they have already been consuming plenty of foods on this list. Increasing the volume of fresh fruits and vegetables that they consume while reducing the intake of processed foods is the best place to start. Take the changes one step at a time so that you can focus on them.

Educate yourself about the reasons why a gluten lifestyle is right for you and get support all around you where you can. Learn about the foods to eat, where you can shop locally, and even online providers that have free or low cost shipping on the items you can't find locally.

Find out about restaurants that offer gluten free meals as well as safe items you can get from standard restaurants. It is possible to live gluten free and to feel very good about your decision to do so. It doesn't have to be expensive and it doesn't have to be difficult.

The good news is that there is more awareness out there about it than in the past. More grocery stores and restaurants are embracing the needs of this sector of consumers. When it comes to what you eat, the choice is always yours.

However, many people in our society today don't eat what they should for their overall health and well-being. With a diet that consists of lots of processed foods you open up the opportunity for serious health problems that can reduce your quality of life and also your overall lifespan.

A gluten free diet isn't going to harm you like many fad diets will out there. This should be encouraging information if you are switching to this type of lifestyle because you want to rather than because you medically have to.

It is never too late to change your habits and start with a gluten free diet that works well for you. This type of diet can work for your entire family and they won't feel like they are missing out on anything! Consider such changes an investment in your quality of life, your longevity, and your opportunity to really lead by example for your children!

It is estimated by 2015 that there will be more than $5 billion annually for sales of gluten free products. This isn't a passing trend, this is a lifestyle change and a way of life for many people. The possibilities continue to grow and that makes it easier to embrace this type of living without difficulty and without it being an expensive endeavor.

Personal Choice

For those with true celiac disease, it must be hard to comprehend why anyone who did not have to would go on a gluten-free diet. Gluten-free products are extremely costly and definitely do taste differently.

Having said that, individuals become gluten-free for many reasons:

1. According to celebrities in the media, it is all the rage right now. Some individuals want to be trendy and follow those trends regardless of the reasoning.

2. Other consumers of gluten-free products say that they feel differently when eating a strictly gluten-free diet. Benefits such as more energy, less bloating, better memory are just a few of the claims made by individuals for going gluten- free.

3. Losing weight is a big motivator. Some individuals have pronounced the most positive effect of going gluten-free is the ability to lose weight and keep it off.

4. Avoiding things such as gas, bloating, cramping, and fatigue are a big bonus, as well.

5. Gaining more mental clarity is something that most everyone both male and female would appreciate obtaining.

For many consumers, eating a diet without gluten simply makes them feel better, whether or not they are reaping any scientifically proven benefits and rewards

To avoid feeling the dreaded bloating often associated with eating gluten-filled foods, people may choose to go gluten-free. Bloat is something everyone experiences, some more than others. Women tend to get hit doubly during their menstrual cycle. So if there is even a slim chance to alleviate some of the gluten related bloating, many will be happy to give a gluten-free diet a try.

About The Author

Ruth Smith has authored different cookbooks that surrounds mainly on how to prepare healthy food without hassle. Ruth was able to unfold different methods and tips that cooking is not an ordeal but rather it is something that we shall enjoy.

In all her books, she always stressed out the importance of cooking healthy food over foods that are readily available in fast foods.